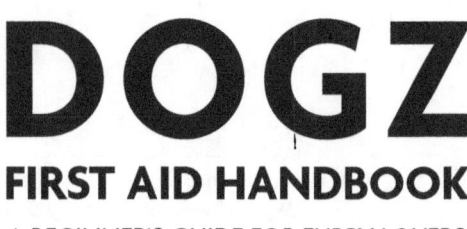

# DOGZ
## FIRST AID HANDBOOK
A BEGINNER'S GUIDE FOR FURRY LOVERS

NEHA PURI & ROHIN BHATIA

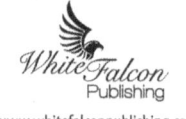

*White Falcon* Publishing

www.whitefalconpublishing.com

Dogz First Aid Handbook
Neha Puri, Rohin Bhatia

www.whitefalconpublishing.com

The contents of this book have been certified and timestamped
on the POA Network blockchain as a permanent proof of
existence. Scan the QR code or visit the URL given on the back
cover to verify the blockchain certification for this book.

The views expressed in this work are solely those of the author
and do not reflect the views of the publisher, and the publisher
hereby disclaims any responsibility for them.

Requests for permission should be addressed to
neha.puri2024@gmail.com

ISBN - 978-1-63640-521-6

Pet first-aid is defined as **the immediate treatment of an animal that is injured or is suffering from sudden illness; it could be at home or during travel or on the road.**

First-aid is only to safeguard the well-being of animals in an emergency. The objective of pet first-aid is to preserve life, to reduce pain and suffering, to prevent the state from getting worse and to stimulate recovery.

Whether you are trying to help your pet dog or a stray that you might come across around you, the basics of first aid remain the same. Most people that spot an injured dog expect an ambulance, NGOs or other animal welfare organisations to reach on the spot and end up wasting time that they otherwise could have used to provide first aid on the dogs in need. Try to make a video of the injured dog the moment you see them troubled so that it can be shared with the veterinarian.

Before you carry out first-aid on your dogs, make sure that it is safe for your pet or the strays around you and yourself. Assessing the situation and keeping a check is very important to ensure no harm is caused to you and everyone around you.

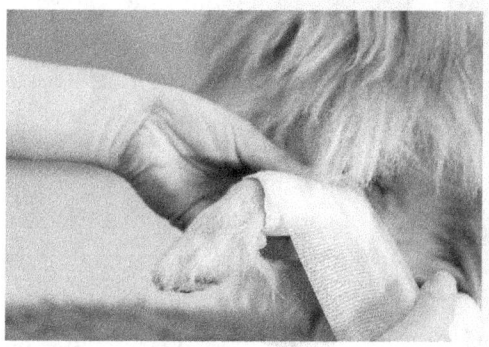

You might often hear how a dog met with a road accident injuring himself and others around him. People generally bypass them thinking it might be dangerous to help those in pain. You must make sure that any action you take will not harm you.

Most importantly, you should be cautious while helping dogs so that they do not bite you or harm you in any way. When your pet or a stray dog is in pain, they might hurt you or bite you because of the pain, and it is very important to understand that precautions are mandatory while dealing with them. At all times, ensure that you are wearing gloves while you are helping the dogs in distress or pain; this is for your own safety. You can only help them if your do not get hurt.

It is important to understand the basics of helping a dog deal with sudden medical emergencies the right way. Our book is here to make you understand the essence of dealing with both your pet dogs as well as the strays who might need medical attention in case of contingency situations.

You never know what might happen when it comes to accidents and

emergencies, so it's good to be prepared. When you're camping, driving across the city or even at home, you need to be ready with the basic know-how to deal with the pets and strays in need.

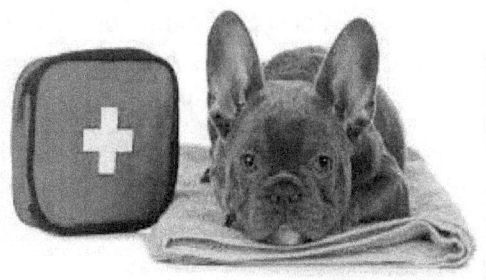

So, we at **DogzKart**, bring you a first-aid guide for your furries. Just like you have a first-aid kit for the humans at your home, it's important to keep one handy for the canines in your life.

The information presented herein will help you handle your pet in emergency situations or minor ailments until you

get them to a veterinary clinic for a thorough examination and further treatment.

The best way to manage an emergency is to be prepared with a plan along with the unconditional love for your pet, which includes having a first-aid kit, having on-hand emergency hospital contact numbers and access to dog ambulances in your area.

In this book, we will take you through the lifestyle of a dog and the way you can help them keep healthy and fit in every age and medical situations. The do's and don'ts while dealing with the canines might save you a lot of time and will guide you to take the right steps at the right time.

We would recommend that you maintain a folder with all the documents and medical history of your pets, any allergies, vaccination details and deworming records.

# SPECIAL THANKS FOR YOUR GUIDANCE DR. SHALLY

This book has been verified and written with the support of our loved veterinarian Dr. Shally Mattoo Jalali. This book would not have been possible without the valuable inputs and research from Dr. Shally who has been a Godmother to my kids with paws: Zoya, Sultan and Karma.

Dr. Shally Mattoo Jalali has an experience of over 14 years in veterinary science, and also holds a Masters in Veterinary Science (Surgery). She pursued her Bachelors in Veterinary Science, A.H and Masters in Veterinary Science (Surgery and Radiology) from Guru Angad Dev Veterinary and Animal Science University, Ludhiana. She has been a Merit holder in the postgraduate programme and has done successful

research work on small animal wound healing and repair.

Dr. Shally started her career with a government job in Punjab, and later, she was one of the founder members and doctors at CGS hospital in Gurgaon. She has also been associated with a lot of NGOs and social causes for strays in India. She is now successfully running SJ's Pet Care Clinic in Gurgaon, Haryana, and have the trust of a lot of pet parents pan India. Her little world revolves around her encouraging parents, supportive husband, amazing daughter Sidhiksha and cutest cat Luna.

# CONTENTS

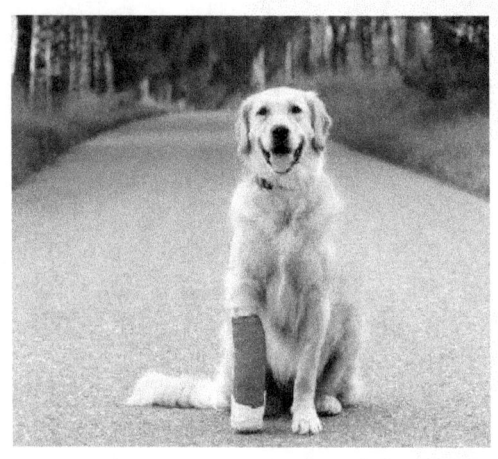

## FIRST-AID ESSENTIALS

## <u>Take a Calming Approach to the Injured Pet</u>

1. Injured or in pain animals become very defensive and aggressive, as they are already in pain. It's better to approach them in a more reassuring way and first calm them down, win their trust and then

help them because if they get hurt
hile you are trying to help them, it
would get even harder for you to
take care of them.

2. Approach your pet in a calming
   tone and sooth them, call them
   with their name or any love
   names you have been calling them
   with.

3. Always muzzle an animal in pain
   or have someone restrain their
   head before examining the injured
   area. This should be taken into
   consideration even with your own
   pet, as all animals can bite when in
   pain.

   **Do not muzzle an animal that
   is having difficulty breathing or is
   vomiting**

4. Try to analyze the nature of the
   emergency as quickly as possible.
   Use the information in this book
   to help stabilize and transport your

pet accordingly. Call a veterinarian as soon as possible and seek professional care for your pet immediately.

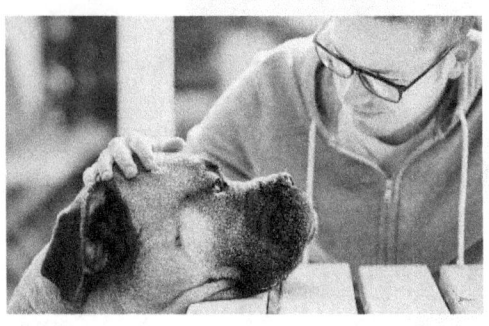

## **First-Aid Kit for Your Pet**

- One first-aid kit pouch – For storage of medicines etc.

- Surgical glove set – To assure that we maintain hygiene while dealing with any dogs

- Gauze sponges – To clean the wounds and cuts

- Cloth muzzle – To prevent your pet from biting you while you are treating them

- Magnifying glass – To concentrate and treat the pet at the exact point of wound

- Tear drops (5 ml) – For the times when your pooch is suffering from any eye infection

- Cotton (15 g) – To clean wounds, soothe wounds and to apply medicines

- Hand sanitizer – To assure your personal hygiene while taking care of your pet

- Digital thermometer – To keep a check on the body temperature of your pet, should be used in the anus of your pet, please assure that your pet does not have an access to the thermometer.

- Crocin drops - To treat fever in your pet. The most commonly used dose rate in dogs is 10 mg/kg orally every 12 hours. NEVER go beyond this does rate without first checking with your veterinarian. Make sure not to use this on cats whatsoever, as Crocin has proven toxic to cats.

- Electrolyte powder (21.8 g x 2) - The pet should be given electrolyte solution orally at the rate of 1/4th cup every half an hour and at least 6-7 cups every 12 hours in case of severe dehydration. It is not advisable if they are vomiting – instead give them small ice chips to lick, which would provide immediate relief to your dogs.

- Medicated wet wipes

- Ointment – To kill and prevent the growth of infection-causing microbes, thereby preventing abrasions, cuts and wounds or

any break in the skin from getting infected. Ensure that your dog does not lick the ointment once applied. An E-Collar is advised to avoid them licking their wounds and the ointments applied, or a bandage should be placed over the affected areas.

- Antihistamine tablets – Primarily, for the management of allergic conditions. Dogs with hypersensitivity to antihistamines should not be given this medicine. Pets with renal or liver problems should be carefully monitored and have their dosages regulated based on the severity of their condition. These medicines have not been proven safe for use in dogs who are pregnant or nursing. This can be taken once a day after consultation from your vet. Their dosage is based off of your dog's overall weight, the ratio being 1 mg of this medicine

per kilogram (dog's weight), while never exceeding the 5 mg cap.

- Tweezers – To extract the unwanted ticks from the fur and body of your dogs

- Topical spray – For any cuts, wounds, allergy or skin problems in your dogs

- Ear drops – These can used when you see your dog scratching its ear often. The dosage rate is 2 drops in a period of 8 hours, repeat if necessary, not more than 4 times without consulting the vet.

- Digestive drops – Generally used on indications of Indigestion, colic, flatulence, intolerance to sudden food changes, Irregular bowel movement and functioning.

- Probiotic powder – To treat diarrhea. This medicine works by restoring the balance of good

bacteria in the intestine that may get upset after antibiotic use or due to intestinal infections.

- Antiemetic medicine – Commonly used to control nausea and vomiting due to certain medical conditions, like upset stomach

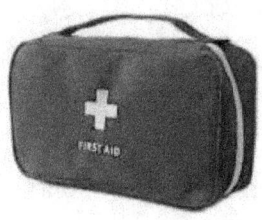

## At-home Medications

Do not give your pet any over-the-counter human medications without checking with a veterinarian first. Many human drugs are toxic to animals and could interfere with medications that a veterinarian would prescribe to help your pet.

## ASSESSMENT OF
## THE CONDITION

### Normal Vital Signs in Your Pet

- Gum color: Generally pink

- Hydration: Pick up skin on nape of the neck of your pet; if it goes back to normal in 5 seconds then your pet is well hydrated.

**For small and medium-sized dogs, normal vitals are as follows:**
Pulse: 70-140 beats per minute
Respiratory rate: 15-30 breaths per minute
Temperature: 100-102.5 °F

**For larger dogs, normal vitals are as follows:**
Pulse: 50-120 beats per minute
Respiratory rate: 15-30 breaths per minute
Temperature: 100-102.5 °F

## Normal Physical Exam of Your Pet

You can quickly analyze your pet's physical condition by watching them and by placing your hands gently in a few body parts of your pet, as discussed below.

**Breathing**: Observe if your pet's chest wall is expanding in and out, slowly and easily. Signs of respiratory distress include an extended head or neck, loud or unusual sounds when breathing, little or no movement of the chest wall when breathing, and an elevated respiratory rate (more than 40-50 breaths/minute when not panting). It is always advisable to make a 5-minute video of your dog while dealing with emergencies, which can be shared with your veterinarian to assess the gravity of the situation.

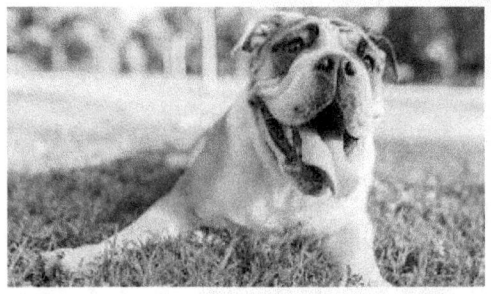

**Heart and circulation:** A pet's normal gum color should be pink. Any other colors of the gums, such as white, lavender, grey or blue, indicates that a pet's blood circulation is not normal. Other indicators that a Pet's heart or blood flow is abnormal include poor or absent pulse and an abnormal heart rate or rhythm.

To check heart rate or pulse, place your hand gently on their inner thigh area and count the number of heart-beats in one minute. Practice this when your pet is at rest so you know what is "normal" for them.

**Temperature:** The only way to take your pet's temperature is through rectal assessment. To take a rectal temperature, lubricate a digital thermometer with petroleum jelly and gently insert the thermometer in the dog's rectum approximately 1–2 inches. The thermometer "beeps" when the accurate temperature is achieved.

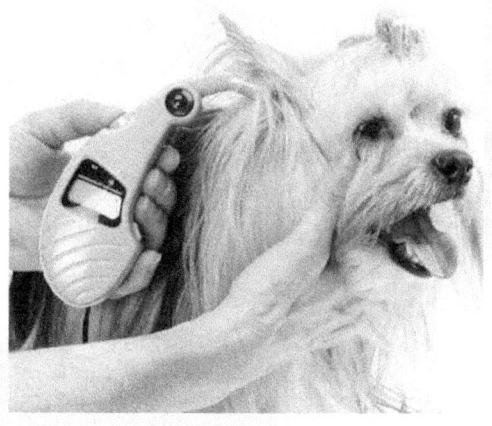

In case of non-cooperative dogs where they do not let you take the rectal temperature at home, go for **axillary**

**temperature** – for which you place the thermometer at 90 degrees into the ear canal of your dog and wait for the thermometer to beep. This temperature may have some variation from the rectal temperature of up to 1 degree. Please note the normal temperature of your dog ranges from **99.5 degrees to 102.5 degrees Fahrenheit**. The third mode to get an idea of high body temperature in your pet is by touching their ear flaps with the back of your hand and if it seems warmer than usual, please go for rectal or axillary temperature measuring process.

**Nervous system:** Watch your pet to make sure they are alert and will interact with you (by voice or touch). Signs that your pet's nervous system is not working fine include restlessness, tremors, seizures, mental dullness, non-responsiveness (stupor or coma) and aimless wandering. Please ensure that you make videos of your pet to share with the veterinarian.

If the nervous system is affected from only the "neck down", then a pet may be lame, weak or unable to walk.

**Abdomen:** Observe on site and touch the area from just behind the rib cage to just before the hind limbs—this is your pet's abdominal cavity. Gently press various parts of their abdomen to locate the exact spot of pain. If your pet is uncomfortable when you touch lower part of their abdomen or ear pinna, that would be the spot where they are feeling the pain. Look for any enlargement of this area and gently press on it to detect any pain. Animals will show these signs when they have problems such as a stomach bloat, a foreign body lodged in their intestines or abdominal bleeding.

**Skin:** The pet's fur can make it difficult for people to see wounds or other problems with their skin. Besides looking at your pet, make sure you

gently run your hands over your pet from "nose to toes" to feel for any pain, wounds, foreign bodies, masses or even insects (i.e., ticks). Gently picking up the skin over the back of your pet's neck is also a good way to assess their hydration level. It should snap back quickly; if the skin stays "tented" even momentarily, it is an indication that your pet is dehydrated and this can quickly become a serious matter of concern.

**Eyes:** When assessing your pet's eyes, have them sit up and look straight forward. The pupils should be equal in size and respond to light by becoming smaller. The whites of the eye should not be yellow, red or discolored and the eyes should be moist and clear. If your pet is squinting, blinking frequently, has unequal pupils, has a large amount of discharge from their eyes, or has blood in or around the eye, they should be taken to a veterinarian immediately.

Splashing eyes with cold water should be done to deal with emergency if you see them frequently blinking their eyes along with other symptoms of eye infections; this would help in clearing off any foreign particles or chemical that could be in their eyes. Please make an immediate video on how they looked like when they were troubled for your veterinarian to get a better understanding.

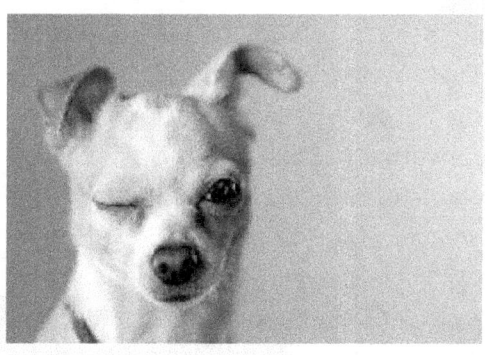

## COMMON DISEASES OF A PUPPY

### Canine Parvo Virus (CPV)

This is a communicable disease and spreads either by direct touch with an infected animal or indirect touch to areas that are contaminated by this virus. Your puppy who is in between the age of 6 weeks to 6 months is most prone to catch parvo virus. It is at risk when it is out and sniffs, licks or consumes infected animal's poop. This virus can stay in the ground soil for up to an year. Take special care when you take your puppy out for a stroll. This virus attacks the puppies in two ways:

a) Intestinal: Signs of vomiting, diarrhea, Loss of appetite and sudden weight loss, lethargy, fever, dehydration, inflammation around eyes and mouth, rapid heartbeat, abdominal pain.

b) Cardiac: Attacks on the heart muscles of young puppies. This is the most lethal form of parvo virus, and sometimes, no symptoms can be seen.

# The life cycle of canine parvovirus

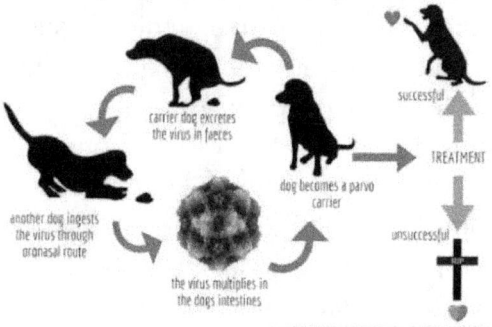

carrier dog excretes
the virus in faeces

successful

TREATMENT

dog becomes a parvo
carrier

another dog ingests
the virus through
oronasal route

unsuccessful

the virus multiplies in
the dogs intestines

If you see any one or more above mentioned symptoms in your dog, then immediately get them tested for parvo virus at your vet's clinic or hospital.

Precautions: Get your pet vaccinated between 6-8 weeks of age followed by booster shots once every year. Before the first vaccination of the puppies, be

cautious about where you take them. This is a serious disease especially in young puppies and can prove fatal if not treated on time and in the correct manner.

Treatment: This infection needs hospitalization of your pet for 3-8 days depending on their situation. An infected pet is kept away from all the dogs in the hospital and regular fluids and medicines are given to him through injections. These include intravenous immunoglobulins for treatment of parvo virus. Dogs are discharged from the hospital after they stop vomiting, are hydrated and start eating willingly, but the at-home total recovery time is estimated to be around 1 month. The vaccinations are only recommended one month after complete recovery from parvo virus Infection. It is advised to keep them away from other pets and public places during the recovery phase to avoid spreading the infection

further. Humans are immune to CPV and are at no risk to get infected.

## Canine Distemper

This is a highly contagious disease caused by the paramyxovirus. It is one of the most common viruses found in dogs and many other animals. Your dogs may get infected through contact with an infected animal's urine, blood, saliva or respiratory droplets, and can also spread through coughing, sneezing and contaminated food and water bowls.

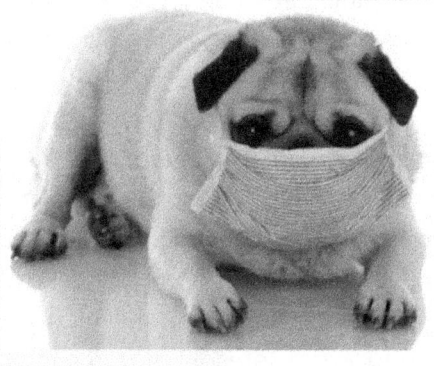

Symptoms: The symptoms for canine distemper takes up to 14 days to show after getting infected. It impacts the gastrointestinal, respiratory, skin, immune and nervous systems. The visible signs in your dog can include fever, difficulty in breathing, coughing, sneezing, lethargy, eye discharge, nasal discharge, vomiting, diarrhea, loss of appetite, swollen nose and foot pads, pneumonia, sores on the skin and pain. These also include some neurological symptoms, such as muscle twitching, seizures, paralysis (or partial paralysis), circling, head tilt, chewing gum fits, excessive salivation and eye movements.

Treatment: Get your dog vaccinated for canine distemper once your puppy is 6 weeks old. Please consult your vet for the follow-up vaccinations as every country has different vaccination circulars and mandates for distemper. Your dog needs to be hospitalized for

the treatment of this virus. There is no particular treatment for distemper in general and treatment is given as per the symptoms and severity of the symptoms. The treatment includes electrolytes, pain relievers, seizure medications, broad spectrum antibiotics, good nutrition and fever reducers. In more severe cases, they might be advised to put on steroids.

Adult dogs can recover from canine distemper, but even after the recovery, they might face a lot of neurological or central nervous disorders, such as brain damage, nerve damage, seizures, jaw spasms and muscle twitching.

## **Kennel Cough**

If your dog constantly makes sounds of choking on something, they may be infected with kennel cough or canine infectious tracheobronchitis. It is also called Bordetella as it is usually caused by the virus of the same name. It is

not usually a serious ailment and most dogs can recover from kennel cough with ease. This disease impacts the respiratory tracts of the canines.

Causes: The most common cause of catching kennel cough is exposure to poorly ventilated conditions, such as kennels for dogs, where they stay in groups.

Treatment: There are three forms of vaccines for kennel cough – intravenous, nasal mist and oral.

## **Adeno Virus**

This virus in dogs causes respiratory infections, attacks multiple organs in a dog's body and causes infectious canine hepatitis (ICH). This ailment attacks the liver and be fatal in 30% of the cases.

Symptoms: Immediately get your pet tested at the vet if you observe any of

the following symptoms and keep your dog hydrated at all times – difficulty in moving one of more limbs, bruising, inflammation of the brain, convulsions, bleeding mouth and gums, small red dots on the skin, jaundice, diarrhea, abdominal pain, vomiting, swelling in the neck and head, increased thirst, bluish cloudy eyes, respiratory infection, discharge from eyes and nose, loss of appetite, fever above 104 °F, and cough.

Treatment: If your pet is tested positive of adeno virus, get them hospitalized immediately. The doctors might have to provide intravenous fluids to keep the dog rehydrated; in more serious cases, blood transfusion is advised too. It is advisable to always get your dogs vaccinated annually, but differs from pet to pet and its vet is the best judge to take a call on its vaccination schedule. Every country has different circulars on the vaccination schedules

and it is always advisable to consult your veterinarian.

## <u>Rabies</u>

Rabies is a vaccine-preventable, zoonotic, viral disease. This is a lethal RNA virus that affects all mammals and dogs and attacks the brain, the spinal cord and the central nervous system. Its causative agent is rabies virus (RV). Rabies is a **viral zoonotic disease** that causes progressive and fatal inflammation of the brain and spinal cord.

While it's preventable and even treatable if caught early on, once the symptoms of rabies appear, the virus is fatal.

*<u>How rabies can spread</u>*

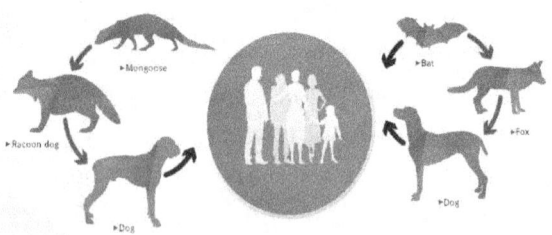

Causes: Rabies virus is secreted in saliva, so it's most often passed through a bite wound from an infected animal. When a bite breaks the skin, the virus can enter the bloodstream. It can also pass through an open wound that is exposed to the saliva of an infected animal, usually by licking.

While it can pass between pets, rabies in dogs most frequently comes from exposure to wild animals like bats, raccoons and foxes.

Symptoms: If your dog is bitten by another animal and you're worried about rabies, pay close attention to their behaviour and call your vet immediately if you have reason to suspect rabies. Your dog may quickly become restless and irritable, even showing aggression. Closely observe the changes - If your dog is usually excited and happy, they may suddenly seem relaxed and disinterested. Physical signs

of rabies in dogs include fever, difficulty swallowing, excessive drooling, staggering, seizures and even paralysis.

As the virus progresses, your dog may act as though they are overstimulated, which means lights, movement and sound may appear to have a negative effect. They may seek out a dark, quiet place to hide or act. One of the most well-known symptoms of rabies in dogs is foaming at the mouth. Some dogs may not show "foaming" but simply excess saliva or drooling. This is a sign that the virus has progressed. In the final stages of rabies, seizures and increasing paralysis are common. Dogs in this stage can't control their muscles — especially in their head and throat — which makes swallowing difficult. Eventually, breathing isn't possible, which leads to death.

The virus can be in your dog's body for weeks before any signs develop. Most

cases in dogs develop within 21 to 80 days after exposure, but the incubation period can be much shorter or longer. Once rabies shows symptoms, it can't be treated, so it's important to call your vet as soon as your dog has been bitten, instead of waiting.

Precautions: Getting your dog vaccinated for rabies is a mandate as per the law in most of the countries. This not only protects your dog from getting infected but also protects the other dogs and humans around in case they bite them. Always make sure to take your dog out for a walk in known and safe surroundings and where there is no threat of his encounter with other animals who would be rabies infected. Even after taking all the precautions if your pet is bitten by another animal, Immediately wear gloves, muzzle your dog and clean the wound with ethanol or other disinfectant available in your pet emergency first-aid kit, calm your

dog and take them to the veterinarian at the earliest for further treatment.

<u>Diagnosis</u>: There's no test to detect the early stages of rabies infection. The rabies virus contaminates the blood stream and shows its presence in the saliva of the animal too. After the onset of symptoms, a doctor can use tests such as a blood, tissue or saliva test to help determine whether your dog have the disease. Tissue tests include the direct fluorescent antibody (DFA) test and a biopsy of the neck.

It is advisable to immediate isolate your dog who has been bitten and is at potential risk of rabies. Get his blood culture and saliva culture done to inspect them for the rabies virus.

If you've been bitten by a wild animal, a doctor will typically administer a preventive shot of the rabies vaccine to stop the infection before symptoms set

in. Immediate medical attention and treatment is recommended for your dog as well anyone in your family to deal with rabies.

## Canine Leptospirosis

This is **an infectious disease that causes serious illness in** dogs, other animals and people. The disease is caused by spiral-shaped bacteria called leptospires that live in water or warm, wet soil. Initial signs of leptospirosis include fever, lethargy and lack of appetite.

Causes: The bacteria that cause leptospirosis are spread through the urine of infected animals and can survive in water or soil for weeks to months. People and animals can get infected through contact with contaminated urine, water or soil. When leptospirosis does cause disease in dogs, it tends to be most severe in unvaccinated dogs that are younger than 6 months of age.

It takes about 4-12 days after exposure for a dog to start to feel ill.

Precaution: It is always advisable to consult your veterinarian to advise when to get the leptospirosis vaccination done for your dog to avoid any ailments in the future, and also follow the booster shots as recommended by your veterinarian. Prevention is best accomplished by stopping your dog's access to contaminated water. Also, try to sanitize your dog's environment by eliminating food and garbage to the minimum.

Leptospirosis is a zoonotic disease and contagious to humans too. The most likely way in which humans contract leptospirosis is via exposure to dog or rat urine. However, any bodily fluid, including vomit and saliva, can transmit the disease. If your dog is infected with leptospirosis, it is very important to practice proper hygiene even after

he has recovered (wearing protective gloves when cleaning up after your dog, preventing face-licking, etc.)

Vaccination for leptospirosis is an option to consider if your dog is at high risk of contracting the disease. The American Animal Hospital Association considers leptospirosis a "non-core" vaccine for dogs. That is, they do not recommend it unless there is a good chance your dog will be exposed to leptospirosis. The efficacy of the vaccine is variable: short-lasting or limited. There have been reports of reactions to the vaccine that vary from minor to severe.

Vaccination does not always prevent infection, but it tends to make the disease much milder if infection occurs. There is the potential for vaccinated dogs that do become infected to become long-term carriers of leptospirosis. Some long-term carriers have more frequent incidence of reproductive failure and stillbirths.

Diagnosis: Blood tests will show changes in kidney or liver parameters. Diagnosis is made through blood and urine tests that look specifically for leptospirosis. Antibiotics are typically used to treat leptospirosis; not only can they treat the active infection, but also prevent dogs from becoming carriers of this virus.

Treatment: Patients with suspected or confirmed leptospirosis should receive a combination of antimicrobial therapy and supportive care tailored to each patient according to severity of clinical signs and affected organ systems.

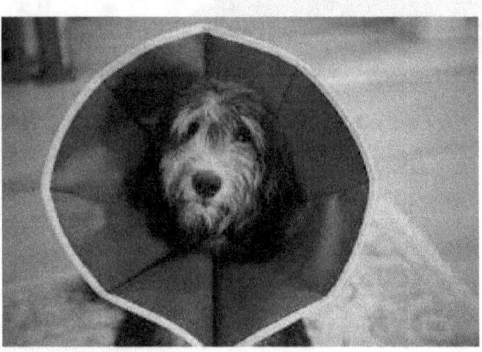

Antibiotic therapy for dogs with leptospirosis are IV penicillin derivatives or oral doxycycline. After gastrointestinal signs have resolved, oral doxycycline should be administered for 2 weeks to clear leptospires from the renal tubules and eliminate the carrier status. The following medications are recommended only under the supervision and presence of a veterinarian:

- Ampicillin 20–30 mg/kg IV q6–8h

- Penicillin G 25,000–40,000 U/kg IV q6–8h

- Doxycycline 5 mg/kg PO q12h or 10 mg/kg PO q24h

Supportive care may be required depending on different levels of the severity of illness and affected organ systems. Recommendations commonly include maintaining adequate hydration with IV fluid therapy; correcting electrolyte and acid-base derangements;

and administering anti-emetics, anti-hypertensives, pain control medications and nutritional support.

## Canine Corona Virus

It is a highly infectious intestinal infection in dogs and specially puppies. Canine coronavirus is usually short-lived but may cause considerable abdominal discomfort for a few days in infected dog and causes gastrointestinal problems in dogs.

Causes: Canine coronavirus are contracted by oral contact with infected faecal matter. A dog may also become infected by eating from contaminated food bowls or by direct contact with an infected dog.

Crowding and unsanitary conditions lead to coronavirus transmission. The incubation period from ingestion to clinical signs is one to four days. The

duration of illness is two to ten days in most dogs. Secondary infections by bacteria, parasites and other viruses may develop and prolong illness and recovery. Dogs may be carriers of the disease for up to six months after infection.

Symptoms: Sudden diarrhea, lethargy and decreased appetite. The stool is loose, with a fetid odor and orange tint. It may contain blood or mucus. If a puppy has a mixed infection, for instance both coronavirus and parvo virus, the illness will be more severe. Immediately take your pet to the veterinarian if you see these signs and start the treatment as directed by them.

Treatment: There is no specific treatment for canine coronavirus and the treatment is given as per the symptoms and the organs and body parts impacted and its severity. Antibiotics are ineffective against viruses, but may

be useful in controlling secondary bacterial infections. Withholding food for twenty-four hours after diarrhea ceases and gradually reintroducing small amounts of food may be the only required treatment. A dehydrated patient may require intravenous fluids to correct the fluid and electrolyte imbalances. Early medical intervention is the key to successful treatment of severe cases.

## Cardiac Discomfort

<u>Signs</u>: Collapse, weakness, bluish or gray gum color, rapid/slow heart rate, increased respiratory rate, coughing, respiratory distress and vomiting.

<u>Action</u>: Call and seek veterinary care immediately. Such emergencies should not be taken lightly as they are often life threatening. Limit your pet's activity; carry them if possible.

## Urinary Infections or Irritants

<u>Signs:</u> Frequent urination or straining, blood in urine, difficulty urinating, vomiting, lethargy, abdominal pain and vocalizing.

<u>Action</u>: Animals can develop urinary blockage and infections similar to

humans. Often straining to urinate can be confused with constipation.

## **Diarrhea/Loose Motions**

Diarrhea can be due to stress, a change in your pet's diet or an underlying medical problem. New food items should be introduced in your pet's diet slowly in small quantities and the switch should be gradual, giving their bodies time to get accustomed with the change. Diarrhea can often be a symptom of a more serious illness or disease. Make sure that your pet continues to drink enough water. If the diarrhea persists for more than 12–24 hours, seek veterinary assistance. The quick hack is to feed some plain yogurt and psyllium husk mix to your pet to provide immediate relief. It is best to feed a pet with diarrhea a bland diet; an example bland diet that works includes plain white rice and white chicken meat (with no skin)

that is fed in small amounts. If your pet is showing other signs of illness (i.e. vomiting/lethargy/weakness) do not wait, seek veterinary attention immediately.

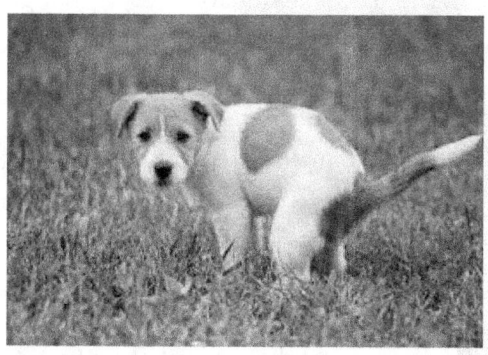

## **Cold Weather**

Dogs with short hair coats, dogs that are left without shelter and dogs exercising in cold weather (or during weather extremes) are more prone to cold stress injuries.

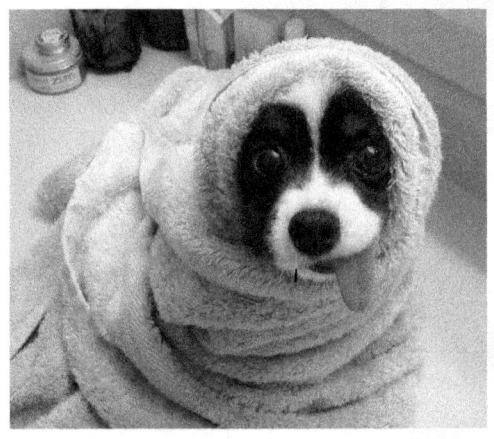

<u>Signs</u>: Shivering, lethargy, weakness, inability to use limbs, pale/blue gums, quiet/dull mentation and rectal temperature of 85-99 °F.

<u>Action</u>: Move your pet to a warm place and wrap them in warm blankets or towels. Do not rub your pet vigorously with the blankets or towels as this can damage cold tissue and make frostbite worse. If the animal is wet and cold, a hair dryer on the warm setting can be used with caution. Try to raise your pet's

body temperature slowly over 30–60 minutes. Warm water bottles (wrapped in towels to avoid direct contact with skin) can be used under the blankets to help increase your pet's temperature. Frost bitten skin can be very painful and fragile. Transport any pets with hypodermic injuries immediately to a veterinary hospital for further care. Do not use electric heating pads, electric blankets or unwrapped hot water bottles in any form.

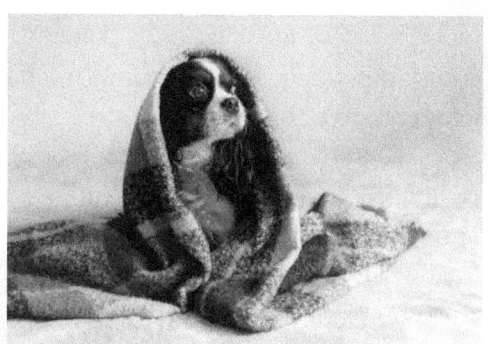

<u>Prevention</u>: Dog hoodies and jackets are made by several companies and are very helpful in preventing cold

weather-related illnesses. Limit the length of time a pet is exposed to rain and extreme cold weather. Make sure that you take care of the hygiene of your dogs while you dress them up. Make sure you remove their clothes every 2-3 days and wash them with disinfectant before you put them on.

## **Shock**

Shock is the condition where there is a lack of oxygen in the body's tissues. This can be from blood loss or problems with distribution of blood in the body. Common emergencies that can cause shock in pets include trauma, bloating, infection, hyperthermia, poison ingestion and severe allergic reactions.

Signs: Pale/white gum color, high or low heart rate (>180 or <60 in a dog), often increased respiratory rate, weak pulses, limbs might feel cool and the pet is quiet and lethargic.

Action: Keep the pet calm and transport immediately to a veterinary clinic. Control all sources of external bleeding with direct pressure. Wrap pets that are cold in warm blankets. A quick home remedy that can help deal with the situation immediately is to give some honey with a pinch of salt. Avoid giving any sedative as it will worsen the condition further.

## Trauma

Any type of injury or accident that occurs to your dog is considered a trauma. Major types of trauma include being hit by a car, getting in a dog fight, falling from a height or experiencing any other traumatic event. Minor injuries are also considered traumas, such as cutting a paw on something sharp or tearing a toenail. Pets that have undergone traumas may experience shock, wounds, broken bones, head trauma, internal injuries and more. Shock is especially common in trauma victims.

<u>Signs</u>: Most animals that undergo trauma are in shock.

- Heart rate and respiratory rate are often high.

- Pets are often dazed and may not respond normally. Many pets may appear to be normal but internal injuries may have occurred.

All animals that experience trauma should be seen by a veterinarian and observed for 12–24 hours.

<u>Action</u>: Keep calm and immediately prepare the pet for transport to a veterinary hospital. Keep the pet warm and apply pressure to any areas with external bleeding.

## **Abdominal Pain or Discomfort**

<u>Signs</u>: Howling, listlessness, restlessness, lethargy, arching back, unable to get comfortable, vomiting, diarrhea, bloated or distended abdomen.

\* Unproductive nauseous retching in a medium to large breed dog is a true emergency.

<u>Action</u>: Do not give your pet food or water — this may induce vomiting and make the condition worse. Abdominal pain can be very serious and is often life-threatening if not addressed as soon as possible. Limit the activity of your pet. You can put small pets in a box or a carrier. Call a veterinarian and seek professional help as soon as possible. Avoid giving any painkillers as they might increase the abdominal pain.

## **Vomiting**

Look for signs of foreign material or strange food that you have not fed your pet in the vomit. When you call the veterinarian, let them know if your pet has eaten any foreign objects or new foods. Rest the stomach for 4–6 hours by offering no food or water. Then, try small amounts of water and bland food every 2 hours.

A bland food diet for pets includes the following: plain white rice and white chicken meat (no skin) for your canines. If the pets eat this bland food well with no vomiting, they can be kept on this diet for 24 hours. After 24 hours, slowly transition them back to their regular food by mixing the bland food and regular diet together (more regular food mixed with less bland food). Look for any foreign body in the mouth – it could be a rope toy or any other article they could be playing with and is stuck in their mouth. They can be given some plain yogurt as it is full of probiotics. If vomiting persists, or your pet has unproductive vomiting (retching) or abdominal distension, see your veterinarian immediately.

## **Gastric Dilatation Volvulus (Bloat)**

This is an absolute emergency! This could occur in any medium- to large-sized, deep-chested dog. Great Danes are the most susceptible breed. Other

breeds commonly affected include Dobermans, German Shepards, Labradors and Weimaraners.

<u>Signs</u>: Nonproductive retching/vomiting, hyper salivation, restlessness, abdominal distension/pain and anxiety.

<u>Prevention</u>: The cause of bloat is unknown but extreme stress (while boarding, flying, etc.) and feeding dogs immediately prior to exercise may increase the incidence of bloating. Bloat is also more likely to occur in deep-chested breeds.

<u>Action</u>: Seek immediate veterinary care. This is a serious surgical emergency and is life-threatening if action is not taken immediately.

A rophylactic gastropexy (minimally invasive surgery) to prevent GDV can be performed on susceptible breeds in severe and emergency situations.

## **Allergic Reactions**

<u>Signs</u>: Fever, vomiting, diarrhea, scratching, chewing at feet, swollen face or puffiness around eyes, troubled breathing, weakness and collapse.

<u>Causes</u>: Allergic reactions can result from a variety of causes, including insect bites or stings, food reactions, environmental issues and vaccines.

<u>Action</u>: Call a veterinarian Immediately. Allergic reactions should be treated immediately to prevent shock. A thorough examination by a veterinarian should still be performed on your pet, even if you see an improvement.

<u>Tip</u>: Vaccines can cause both mild and severe allergic reactions in pets. Some of these reactions can happen immediately and others within hours (or days) of taking vaccine. If your pet has a history of vaccine reactions, discuss

this with your regular veterinarian; altering the vaccine protocol may be recommended.

## **Insect Bites**

Just like humans, animals vary in their reactions to insect venom.

<u>For small local reactions</u>, there is swelling and pain at the sting site but no other clinical signs. Try to remove stinger while keeping the pet calm, clean the site and then apply ice. Monitor your pet closely for the next several hours to make sure no further swelling or breathing problems occur.

<u>For large local reactions</u>, where there is swelling of the face, a limb or "hives" all over the body, keep the pet calm and transport them to a veterinary facility immediately. These are called anaphylactic shocks.

Severe life-threatening toxic reactions occur when a pet is the victim of multiple stings at once in case of getting directly exposed to a beehive. First and foremost, do not put yourself between a pet and a swarm of bees or wasps. If the swarm is still present, have trained personnel wearing full safety gear rescue the pet. Once the majority of insects have left the victim, throw a blanket over the pet and transport them to a veterinary facility immediately.

## **Bite Wounds**

Signs: The appearance of wounds and skin trauma may vary from injury to injury, but redness, swelling and dirt inside the wound are common features.

Action: Approach the animal slowly. Muzzle the animal or have someone restrain the head. Examine the entire animal for bleeding, bite wounds or pain. Multiple bite wounds can be hard to find under thick fur.

Flush each bite wound with saline water, soap or disinfectant, and transport the pet to a hospital for further care. Bite wounds are very prone to becoming infected and your pet should be examined for signs of infection and further injury deep in the wound. Wrap large wounds for transport; small wounds can be left uncovered. Seek immediate veterinary care if your pet gets bitten by a snake or spider.

## Bleeding Wounds/Lacerations

Approach the animal slowly and muzzle your pet as the first step. Remove dirt and debris from around the wound and wash the wound with clean water or saline solution. Do not apply anything harmful into the wound like soap or hydrogen peroxide. Use firm pressure, if needed, to stop bleeding. Apply direct pressure to bleeding wounds with gauze or a clean towel/cloth. Wrap large wounds prior to transport;

small wounds can be left uncovered. If your pet has an impalement injury (penetration with a foreign object, like a stick, arrow, etc.), do not remove the object. Help stabilize the object close to the area of penetration and transport the pet immediately to an emergency hospital.

## **Burns**

Signs: A pet's fur may be scorched and their skin can often initially be red and inflamed. Inflamed skin progresses over time to open wounds with discharge.

Action: If you see that your pet has gotten burned (i.e., due to accidental spillage of extremely hot fluids) or see evidence of a burn, immediately flush the area with normal water for 5–10 minutes. After flushing, apply a cool, wet compress to the injured area. *Never apply an ice pack or ice

directly to an animal's skin*. Apply honey locally on the burned part.

Call a veterinarian and seek professional help; your pet's skin can be severely burned but difficult to assess because it is thicker than a human's and covered with fur. Burns need to be taken care of immediately and can be life-threatening when severe.

## Fractures

<u>Signs</u>: Pain, not using a limb or a limb looking abnormally bent or swollen.

<u>Action</u>: Muzzle the animal or have someone restrain the head. Check the limb for open wounds or bleeding. If the wound is bleeding excessively, apply pressure with a towel or other available (clean) cotton material and try not to move the limb. Do not pull on the limb in an attempt to align the fracture; such action can result in further injury and increased bleeding.

Stabilize the limb if possible. Magazines, newspapers, etc. can be used as splints for support but incorrect placement of a splint can lead to further injury. Carry your pet, if possible, to prevent weight bearing on the limb and seek professional help. Do not give any pain medications to your pet (as some are toxic to animals) unless instructed to do so by a veterinarian. Avoid wrapping the leg (unless large wounds are present) as it is easy to impede blood circulation. Ice packs can also provide immediate relief.

## Seizures

<u>Signs</u>: Shaking (uncontrollably), tremors, strange facial movements, inability to stand, paddling (swimming action) with paws, loss of bowel or urinary control, or acting distant or unresponsive to voice or touch.

<u>Action</u>: Do not try to restrain your pet during an episode. Keep your hands

away from your pet's mouth. Honey mixed with butter can be given orally at home for immediate help.

## Ear Infection

Signs: Scratching at ears, shaking head, whining, head tilting, swollen/puffy ear flaps, strange odor or discharge from ear(s).

Action: Try to prevent your pet from scratching at their ears or shaking their head excessively as this can make the problem worse. Take your pet to a veterinarian to perform a full scan of the inside and the outside of the ear.

## Eye Infection

Signs: Squinting, discharge/tearing, redness, swelling, bleeding and different pupil size.

Action: First step should be to muzzle your dog and then help with the

situation. If there is an obvious wound or foreign object in or around the eye, seek veterinary care immediately. Do not try to bandage the bruising or remove the object. If the source of the irritation is known to be a chemical or fine debris/dirt, flush the eye(s) with sterile saline (or clean water) immediately for 5 to 10 minutes and then seek veterinary care. Eye injuries and infections can get worse very quickly. Immediate medical attention is critical in order to preserve your pet's eyesight.

## **Respiratory Problems**

<u>Signs</u>: Collapse, weakness, blue or gray gum color, labored, rapid or shallow breathing, coughing, anxiety, vomiting and wheezing.

<u>Action</u>: Call and seek veterinary care immediately. Keep yourself and your pet calm. Ensure that the pet is in a cool environment during transport and

do not give anything orally. Difficulty in breathing can result from many conditions, including heart failure, lung disease and/or blockage of the airways.

Such emergencies should be taken seriously as they are often life threatening. If there is a recent history of your pet chewing/swallowing something and you are suspicious that they are choking, use caution and look in your pet's mouth for any foreign object that may be obstructing the airway. Only try to remove the object if it is easily reachable. Any exam of the oral cavity must be done with caution, as bite injuries to you are possible as your pet is already in panic.

## Neurologic

Signs: Inability to use limb(s), inability to stand, circling, seizures, head tilt, abnormal behavior and tremors.

<u>Action</u>: Seek veterinary care as soon as possible. Neurologic disease is difficult to treat and is often quite serious. If your pet is unable to walk, carry them to the car. If they are too big to carry, use a towel (under the abdomen, in front of rear legs) to support the hind end or use a heavy blanket as a stretcher to carry them to the car. Professional diagnosis and treatment is recommended as soon as possible.

<u>Prevention tip</u>: Possible toxins that can cause neurological signs (tremors/seizures) include moldy walnuts, mushrooms, compost, snail and slug bait.

## **Heat Stroke**

Dogs are more susceptible to rapid changes in climate conditions and overheating than humans. They sweat ineffectively and rely on panting to evaporate their body heat. Dogs with

shorter faces (i.e., English and French bulldogs, Pugs, Boxers), dogs with thick hair coats (i.e., Akita, Husky) and dogs with underlying medical conditions or who are obese are at an increased risk of heat exhaustion injury.

<u>Signs</u>: Excessive panting or salivation, lethargy, inability to stand, weakness, lack of coordination, vomiting, diarrhea, bright red tongue/gums, disorientation. If the body temperature is more than 105 °F, then it is a sure matter of concern.

<u>Action</u>: Following are a few of the measures to be taken in cases of heat-related discomfort in your pets:

- Move your pet out of the direct sun to a shady area as soon possible and keep them calm.

- Do not try to get them to stop panting as this is how they cool themselves.

- Gently spray or apply cool, tepid water to the overheated dog. Do not use ice water, ice baths or apply ice to an overheated dog. You can also apply wet, cool towels along the dog's chest, abdomen, between its legs and around the neck. Once cooling measures are initiated, monitor the dog's rectal temperature every 2-3 minutes. Once the body temperature has decreased to 103-104 °F, stop active cooling measures.

- Encourage an overheated dog to drink water but do not force them to drink.

- Air conditioning and fans are also both effective ways to cool an overheated dog.

- Apply alcohol/spirit on foot pads to promote vascular dilation.

Once initial cooling measures have been started, seek veterinary care

immediately. Dehydration of any cause can lead to shock or organ damage. Temperatures of above 105.5 °F in your pet can be life-threatening. Also, light-colored animals can get sunburned just like people. Ask your veterinarian for a recommended sunscreen for your pet.

## Leech Removal

Leeches are a type of parasitic worm that you might encounter in grasses and fresh water. These creatures can attach themselves to humans and feed on their blood. Leeches can also expand up to 10 times their size while feeding, allowing them to consume a lot of your blood at one time. Following a few simple steps that can help you calmly and safely remove a leech without any pain or complications from the bite:

1. **Locate the head and mouth.** A leech's head is smaller and slimmer

than the rest of its body. Look for the narrowest part of the leech to locate its mouth. This is usually the part attached to your pet's coat.

2. **Pull the skin under the leech taut.** Use one hand to gently pull your pet's skin under the leech until it's taut.

3. **Slide a fingernail underneath the mouth.** Gently use tweezers to puncture the leech and put it under the leech's mouth to separate it from your pet's skin.

4. **Flick the leech away.** Use your tweezers to flick the leech away before it reattaches.

5. **Clean the wound.** Clean your pet's wound with rubbing alcohol or a first-aid cleanser to help avoid infection.

6. **Bandage your wound.** You'll see a lot of bleeding when you remove

the leech. Clean the wound and then use a bandage to cover it. Change the bandage frequently for the first few hours until the bleeding stops.

## POISONING

Here are some symptoms that your pet might show if they have ingested a poison:

1.  Weakness

2.  Disorientation

3.  Vomiting

4.  Tremors

5.  Seizures

6.  Salivation (excessive)

If you witness your pet ingesting a poison or if you suspect your pet has been poisoned, call a veterinarian immediately. If the source of the poisoning is known, keep the container beside you while calling the veterinarian as information on the packaging is important in order to determine the

appropriate treatment. If the source is unknown and your pet is showing suspicious symptoms, seek veterinary care for your pet immediately. Treatment to restrain the effects of the poison should be started as soon as possible. If possible, bring the suspected toxic agent with you to the doctor.

## Toxins

Outlined below are several items commonly found in many households that are toxic to pets and the clinical signs pets will show when they have ingested them. Make certain that these items are removed from areas to which your pet has access. If your pet has ingested these products (or is suspected of ingesting these products and is showing the symptoms outlined below) transport them to a veterinarian immediately. Remember to bring the suspected toxic agent with you to the veterinary clinic.

<u>Antifreeze (ethylene glycol)</u>: Pets love the sweet taste! The ingestion of a small amount can be fatal as the antifreeze will cause nervous system and kidney damage. Signs of poisoning include staggering, lethargy, excessive drinking and seizures. An antidote exists but must be given within hours after ingestion to be effective and save a pet's life.

<u>Snail and slug bait</u>: Snail bait is **highly toxic** and even small amounts are enough to cause poisoning in dogs. It can cause life threatening signs in your pet. Signs include nervousness, hyperexcitability, drooling, tremors, rapid heart rate and seizures.

<u>Chocolate</u>: Chocolate (especially semi-sweet, dark, bittersweet and baker's chocolate) and cocoa powder all contain a substance that is toxic to dogs. If ingested, these items can cause nervous stimulation, tremors, rapid heart rate and seizures.

<u>Rat poisons</u>: Some rat poisons cause bleeding, whereas others cause severe brain damage. Since some of these poisons have a delayed effect, you may not see signs that your pet has been poisoned for 3-5 days. If your pet is bleeding from the mouth, nose or rectum or is weak or disoriented, transport them (don't forget the package of suspected toxin!) to the veterinarian immediately.

<u>OTC pain relievers</u>: Human pain reliever pills can cause red blood cell and liver damage, kidney damage, and some salts can cause gastrointestinal problems and bleeding disorders and central nervous system problems in your pets. At all cost, avoid giving any kind of painkillers to your pets unless prescribed by their vet.

<u>Raisins/Grapes</u>: Even small amounts of these products can cause kidney damage or kidney failure in your pet.

<u>Onions</u> (also scallions, onion soup mix, garlic, Allium bulbs): These can cause red blood cell destruction and anemia if consumed by pets.

<u>Xylitol</u>: This is a sugar-free sweetener being used in an increasing number of human products, from chewing gum to pudding to baked goods. Even small amounts of xylitol can cause dangerously low blood sugar levels and liver damage in dogs. Symptoms include vomiting, weakness, abdominal discomfort, collapse and seizures.

<u>Topical flea and tick products</u>: Consumption of OTC flea and tick products typically contain permethrins, which can lead to tremor, twitch, drool and even seizure. These products are only meant for topical application and you should always make sure you keep them away from any kind of access from the pets.

Alcohol: Symptoms of alcohol poisoning in animals are similar to those in people, and may include vomiting, breathing problems, coma and, in severe cases, death.

Avocado: You might think of them as healthy, but avocados have a substance called persin that can act as a dog poison, causing vomiting and diarrhea.

Macadamia nuts: Dogs may suffer from a series of symptoms, including weakness, overheating and vomiting, after consumption of macadamia nuts.

Plants: There are many plants that are potentially toxic to pets. Some cause only mild gastrointestinal upset, whereas others can cause severe organ damage. Just a few of the common plants that may be toxic to pets include:

- Easter Lily, Tiger Lily, and many other Lily species: All parts of the

plant can cause life-threatening kidney damage to pets

- Rhododendron/Azalea: Can cause upset, slow heart rate and shock

- Sago Palm (house plant): Can cause drooling, vomiting and liver failure

- Dumbcane, Dieffenbachia (house plants): Can cause intense burning and swelling of mouth and tongue

- Mistletoe: Can cause vomiting, diarrhea and liver damage

- Castor Beans: Can cause severe gastrointestinal upset, shock and death

- Daffodils, hyacinth, amaryllis, and other bulb plants: Can cause drooling, vomiting, abdominal pain and diarrhea

- Delphinium and Monkshood: Can cause gastrointestinal upset, tremors, seizures and death.

If you have a question as to whether or not a plant is toxic for your pet, contact your local veterinarian.

## Salmon Poisoning

This toxicity in raw salmon can carry an infectious organism (rickettsia) that can cause illness in pets.

Signs: Fever, lethargy and bloody diarrhea. Signs often appear 5–7 days after ingesting a raw fish or parts of a raw fish.

Action: Avoid feeding dogs raw salmonid-type fish (such as salmon, trout or steelhead). Seek immediate veterinary advice if your dog ingests raw fish.

## <u>Dog Park Etiquette</u>

1. Always observe all posted dog park rules.

2. Never leave your dog unattended and watch them closely while they are playing.

3. Be sure your dog is current on vaccines, treated for fleas, dewormed and their medical papers are up-to-date.

4. Always clean up after your dog; carry a poop scooper with you.

5. Do not take puppies younger than 4 months or any dog that is not fully vaccinated to a dog park.

6. If your dog becomes unruly or plays too rough, leash the dog and leave immediately.

7.  If you take children to the dog park, supervise them closely.

8.  Always carry the first-aid kit with you to deal with unplanned emergencies.

## Leaving Your Pet at Home While Traveling

Make a medical records book for your pet and explain the pet-sitter of any allergies and do's and don'ts about your dog.

If someone is taking care of your pet while you are away be in touch with them over video calls, that will make your pet feel your presence. Make certain the pet-sitter is aware of any health issues and veterinary care in case of an emergency.

Always keep first-aid kit at home and explain your pet-sitter how to use the contents of the first-aid kit in case of an emergency.

## **Traveling with Your Pet**

1. Have your veterinarian examine your Pet prior to traveling to make sure it is physically fit to travel.

2. Familiarize yourself with any pet-related restrictions or requirements imposed by airlines, hotels and destination sites prior to traveling.

3. Remember to pack your pet's food and supplies (leashes, medications, water dishes, bedding and litter).

4. Make certain that your pet is wearing identification tags at all times in case he or she becomes lost.

5. Permanent identification microchips that are injected under the pet's skin are available from most veterinarians. Also carry a photo of your pet with you. Bring this emergency booklet, a first-aid kit

and the phone number of your veterinarian in case an emergency should arise.

6. Pets riding inside cars with people should wear seat belts or be secured in a crate. A pet can hurt themselves or other passengers in the car if you slam on the brakes. The safest place to secure your dog is in the middle of the back seat as front-seat air bags can be dangerous for pets.

7. Pets should not be allowed to stick their head out of a car window as flying debris can damage their eyes, ears, face or neck.

8. Pets should never be transported unrestrained on the outside of a vehicle, like the bed of a pickup truck.

9. Never leave your pet unattended in a parked car especially on hot days when heat stroke can occur.

10. When you arrive at your destination, evaluate your pet for illness or injury. Seek veterinary advice immediately if something seems wrong.

11. At all times, carry a first-aid kit, grooming kit and travel kit with you to make the travel seamless and enjoyable for you as well as the pet.

## Skunk Odor Removal

<u>Signs</u>: Potent smell and burning of the eyes.

<u>Action</u>: Put on goggles or other eye protection.

In a bucket, mix:

- 1 quart of 3% hydrogen peroxide

- ¼ cup baking soda

- 1 teaspoon of hand-safe dishwashing liquid

Stir ingredients briefly. The solution will fizz as the hydrogen peroxide decomposes and releases bubbles of oxygen. Have a second person hold the pet in a washtub while you scrub in the solution with a soft brush. Rinse the pet with tap water, taking care not to get this solution into the pet's eyes.

## Tick Removal

When returning from a park or a hike, check thoroughly for ticks by running your fingers through your pet's entire coat, and inspecting the paws, pads, between toes and inside of their ears.

If you find a tick, act in accordance with the following steps:

1. First of all, wear gloves and muzzle your pet.

2. Grab the tick's mouthparts against the skin using tweezers (Do not use your fingers.).

3.  Pull back slowly and steadily with firm force. Do not pull back sharply as this may tear the mouthparts. If mouthparts remain imbedded in the skin, don't panic as mouthparts alone cannot transmit disease. They can, however, act like a splinter and cause an infection, so it is best to remove them.

4.  Do not squeeze or crush the body of a tick or apply substances such as petroleum jelly, alcohol or mineral oil as these may agitate the tick and cause it to inject infective fluids at the wound site.

5.  Following removal of the tick, clean the tick-bite wound, your hands and the tweezers with a disinfectant. Dispose of the tick by placing it in a small sealed container containing alcohol. Once the tick is dead, dispose of the tick and the alcohol by flushing it down the toilet.

## **Fire Safety with Pets**

Millions of pets are affected by house fires every year throughout the world.

The following recommendations are to help pet owners avoid getting their pets to deal with this unfortunate situation:

- Update your home to newer smoke detectors and place them outside each room.

- When you are leaving the house, keep leashes, collars and harnesses near the door and position your dog carriers and kennels near entrances where either you or a fire fighter can easily access them.

- The majority of home fires start in the kitchen. Do not let pets into areas when cooking is in process.

- Place a window cling near the entrance to your house that states

the number of pets in your home and where they are located so that the firefighters and rescuers can do their job quickly.

- Make sure you have at least one working fire extinguisher placed on each floor of your home.

## General Pet Care Tips

1. Avoid over-the-counter flea and tick products; consult your veterinarian for recommendations for safer products.

2. Going out of town? Make sure that your pet-sitter or kennel has written permission to transport your pet to a veterinarian for treatment, if necessary. Also make sure they are updated on current health problems of the pet, their history of allergies and the name/location of your pet's veterinarian.

3. Monitor your pet closely with any chew toys, rawhides, etc. They can potentially swallow large pieces of these toys and this could cause a choking injury or intestinal obstruction.

4. Avoid feeding table scraps to your pets. Rich and fatty foods, in particular, can be very harmful to pets, often leading to vomiting and, possibly, pancreatitis.

5. Try to avoid having your pet drink from standing bodies of water, such as ponds, ditches etc. A very toxic algae (cyanobacteria) can form a green film on the top of still bodies of water, which can be lethal to pets if ingested.

***"Provided what is done, is done in order to save an animal's life or to stop its pain or suffering and is done as an interim measure until a veterinary surgeon's services can be obtained, it is***

*unlikely that, in most cases, there will be subsequent argument that what has been done has gone beyond first-aid."*

This book is intended to help you prevent and deal with pet-related emergency situations that can arise anytime and anywhere. Please assure that it should not be considered as a replacement for the professional veterinary care at any cost.

# DOGZ

## FIRST AID HANDBOOK